I Can Be a Hero

My Grandpa is Extra Sweet:
Diabetic Emergencies

By Leeza Wilson

Printed in the United States of America.
Published by Tsarina Press

Photos courtesy of Pixabay, One Touch, and by permission of Sevier County Ambulance Service and Walden's Creek Fire Department.

ISBN: 978-1-948429-04-7

Legal Disclaimer

Even though I am a licensed EMT Advanced and firefighter, I am not your personal EMT. The information in this book is completely factual, however, for simplicity not all information pertaining to recognition and treatment of a diabetic emergency is relayed in this book. This book should not be used in lieu of seeking advanced medical help in an emergency. If you or a family member, friend, neighbor, or stranger in your presence is experiencing a medical emergency you should call 911.

Dedication

This book is dedicated to my father David M. Knotts
(3/27/36–3/1/17), who had diabetes, and my son Hunter,
who at an early age showed his ability to help take care of
his grandpa and inspired me to write this series. This
series is dedicated to all the little heroes out there that
have stepped up and saved a life and to the emergency
workers and first responders who daily sacrifice their
time, energy, and personal safety to save the lives of
strangers. Special thanks to Sevier County Ambulance
Service, Waldens Creek Fire Department, and One Touch
Diabetic Testing Supplies for the support and permission
to use photos.

Books in this Series

My Grandpa is Extra Sweet: Diabetic Emergencies

The Germ Squad: Colds, Flu, and Stomach Viruses

Where is Your Heartbeat?—Cardiac Emergencies (coming soon)

Preface

This book is part of a series of books that helps teach little children about different types of medical problems and emergencies and what they can do to help their friend or loved one. This story is based on a true story. As an EMT and firefighter, I know how serious a medical emergency can be and how much time matters.

This series of books is designed to help children and their parents or guardians recognize the signs and symptoms of a medical emergency, know when it is appropriate to call 911, and what to do to help someone who is sick or injured while more advanced medical aid is on the way. This series of books is not intended to take the place of more advanced medical aid.

Never underestimate the ability of a young child to understand the medical conditions of family members and close friends and their ability to save a life. Many a child, including my son, have proven their ability to be little life savers and heroes.

Go over this book carefully with your child. Take the time to answer any questions they may have. If someone in your family suffers from a medical condition, such as diabetes, and you feel your child is old enough and mature enough to understand, explain to your child the purpose of the needed medical equipment and when appropriate, how to work it if an emergency should arise in your absence. And please do not forget to explain to your child that medical equipment is not a toy and should never be played with.

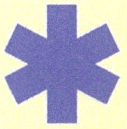 # I Can Be a Hero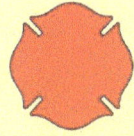

My Grandpa
is
Extra Sweet

Diabetic Emergencies

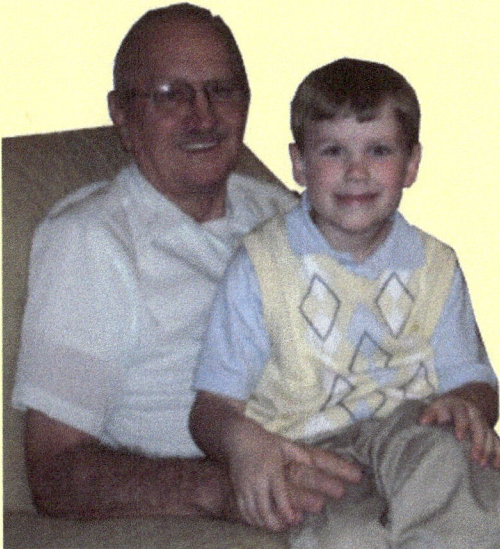

Hi! My name is Hunter. I'm six years old. This is my grandpa. He has **diabetes**. **Diabetes** is an illness that causes his body not to get rid of sugar in his blood like it's supposed to. That means that sugar builds up in his body and makes him sick

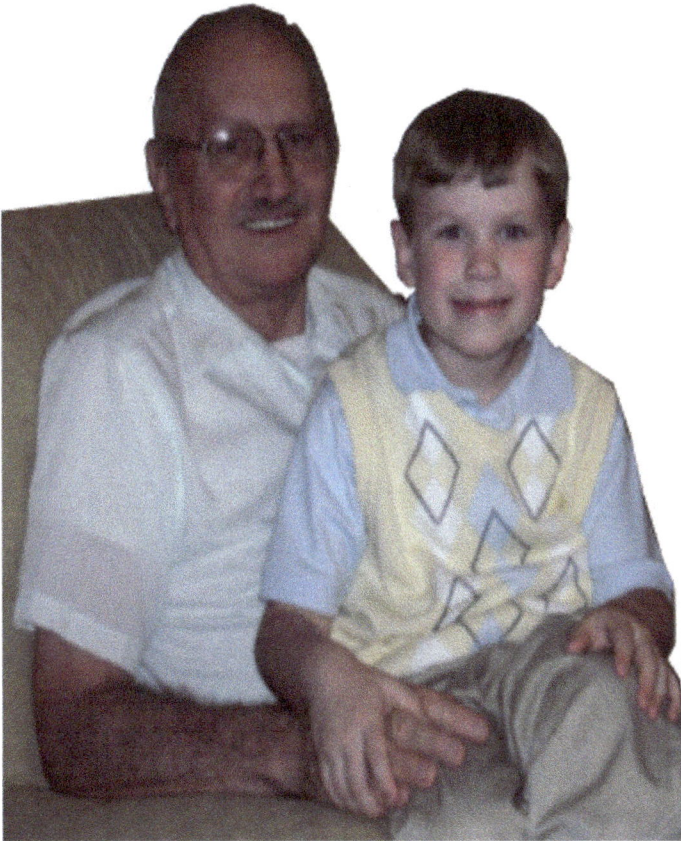

Sometimes grandpa's sugar is too high and. sometimes his sugar is too low. People who have diabetes are called diabetic.

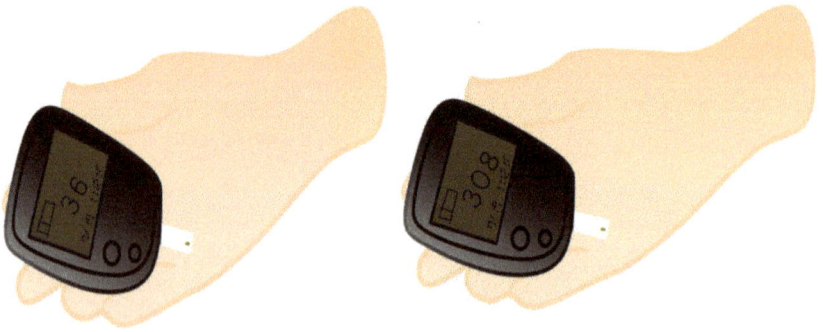

If a **diabetic's** blood sugar gets too low or too high they could die. So **diabetics** have to follow a special diet low in **carbohydrates** and sweets to keep their sugar levels stable.

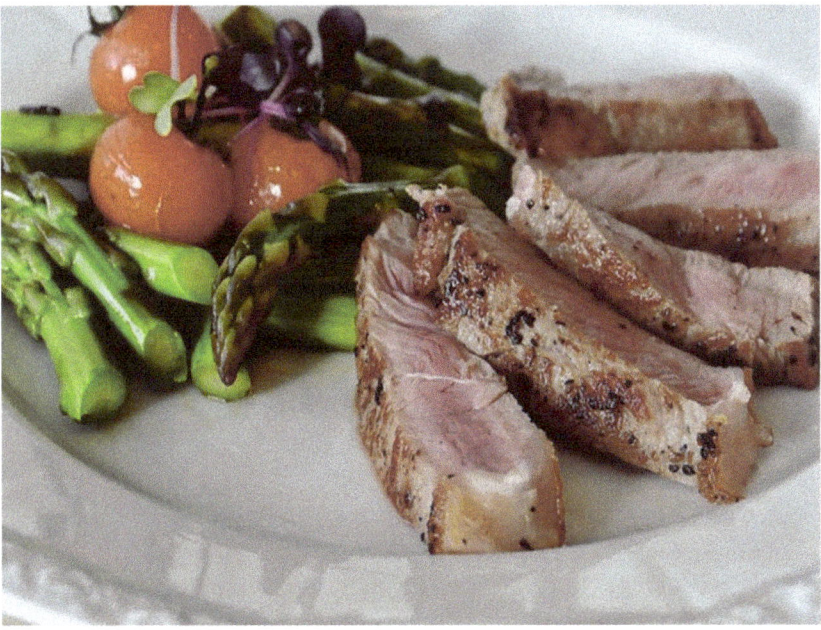

Grandpa has to check his sugar several times a day. To check his sugar, he uses a small machine called a **glucometer**.

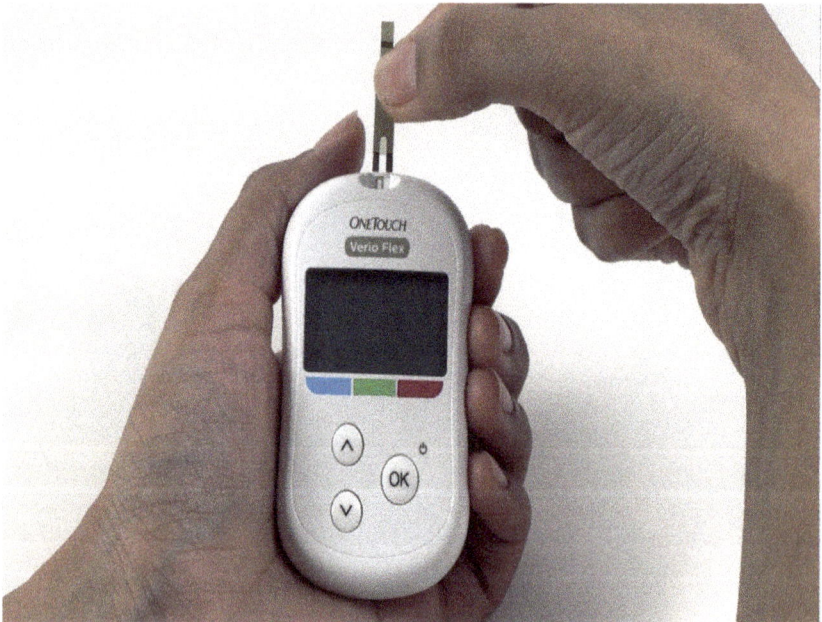

Grandpa puts a small strip with a sensor on the end into the **glucometer**. Then he pricks the end of one of his fingers with a very tiny needle. He squeezes a drop of blood onto the strip. Then the meter tells him what his sugar level is.

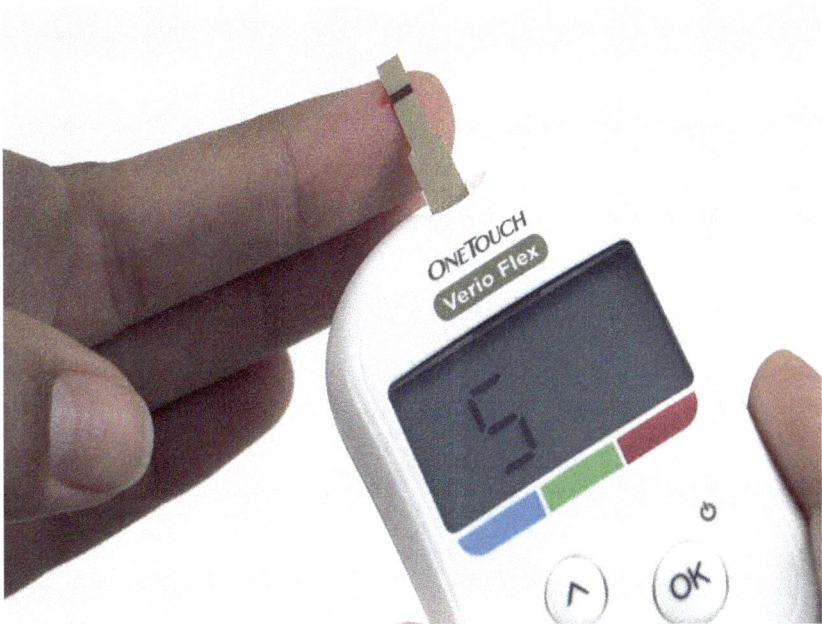

Grandpa has to take a special medicine called **insulin**. **Insulin** is a liquid medicine given as a shot in the skin to lower blood sugar. Some diabetics only need to take a pill to control their blood sugar levels.

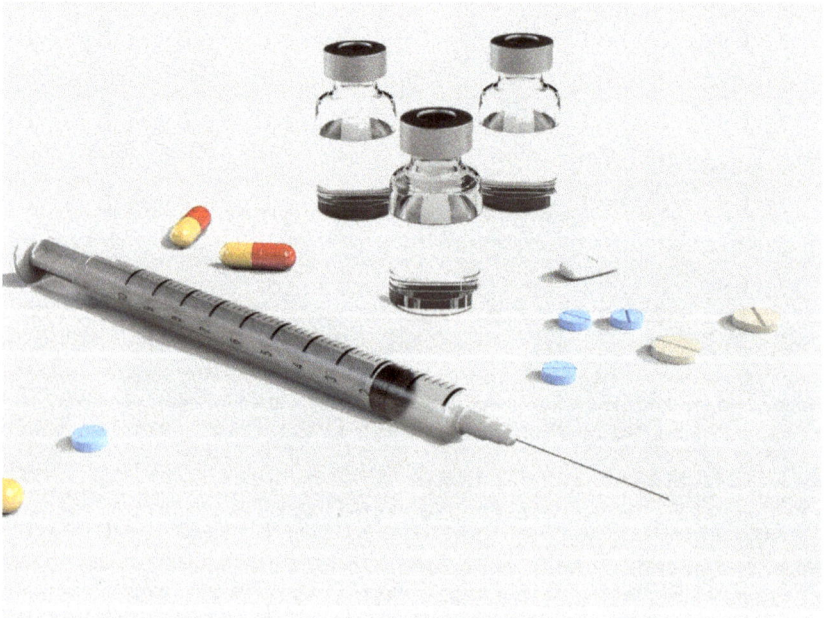

Sometimes when grandpa's sugar is too high his breath smells sweet and fruity, his mouth gets dry, he gets very sleepy, and he is very thirsty.

Then grandpa drinks a lot. That makes him have to go to the bathroom often. If grandpa's sugar gets too high he could have a stroke or go into a diabetic coma.

A diabetic coma means he wouldn't be able to wake up. So when his sugar gets too high it is very important that he take his **insulin.** He also needs to drink a lot a water to flush out the extra sugar.

When grandpa's sugar gets too low he gets very sleepy. He has trouble standing or walking. And his vision may get blurry. His speech gets slow and draggy. And sometimes he shakes and gets very sweaty.

When grandpa's sugar is low and he goes to sleep it is very hard to wake him up.

Sometimes I stay with my grandpa when my mommy is working. One time grandpa's sugar dropped really low. He was having a hard time staying awake.

But grandma, grandpa, and mommy had shown me what to do. I went and got grandpa's **glucometer** and brought it to him. I called him in the loudest voice I could use. That woke him up him enough to check his sugar.

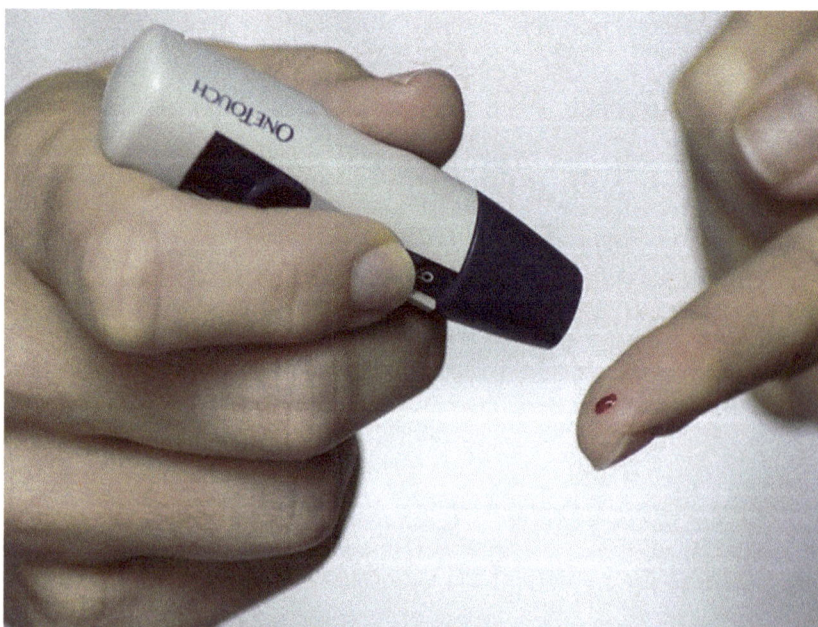

A normal blood sugar should be above 80 and below 120. Grandpa's blood sugar was 43. I knew grandpa needed orange juice and something to eat to bring his sugar level up.

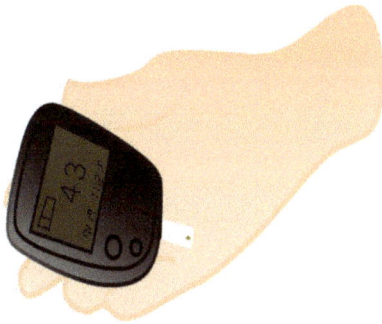

I got grandpa a glass of orange juice. I made sure he was alert enough that it was safe for him to swallow without choking. I helped him stay awake to drink his juice. Soon grandpa was feeling better.

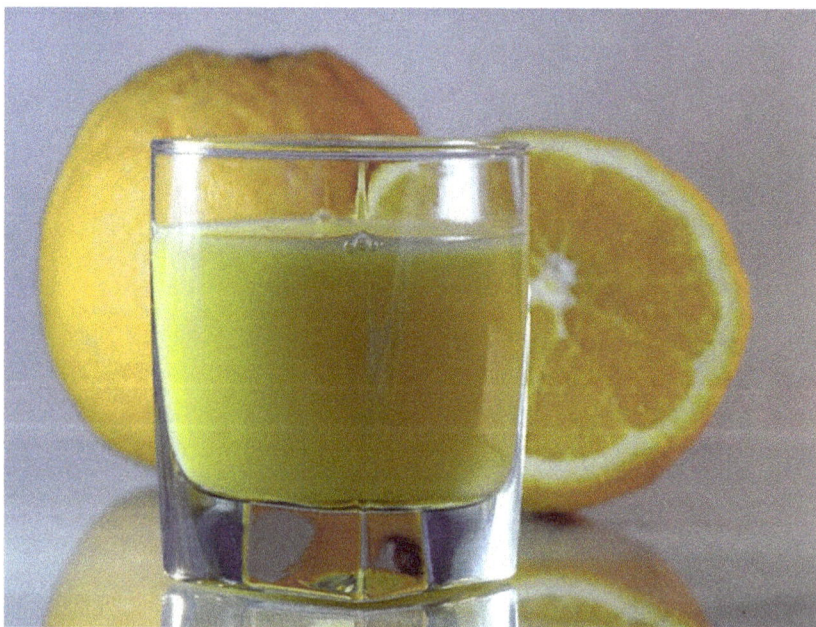

You should never force anyone who is not fully awake to eat or drink anything. It could cause them to choke or accidentally breathe the food or drink into their lungs.

After grandpa was feeling a little more alert we went to the kitchen and had a peanut butter snack. After that, grandpa checked his sugar again. It was above 80. Grandpa was a lot more alert now and his speech was much clearer.

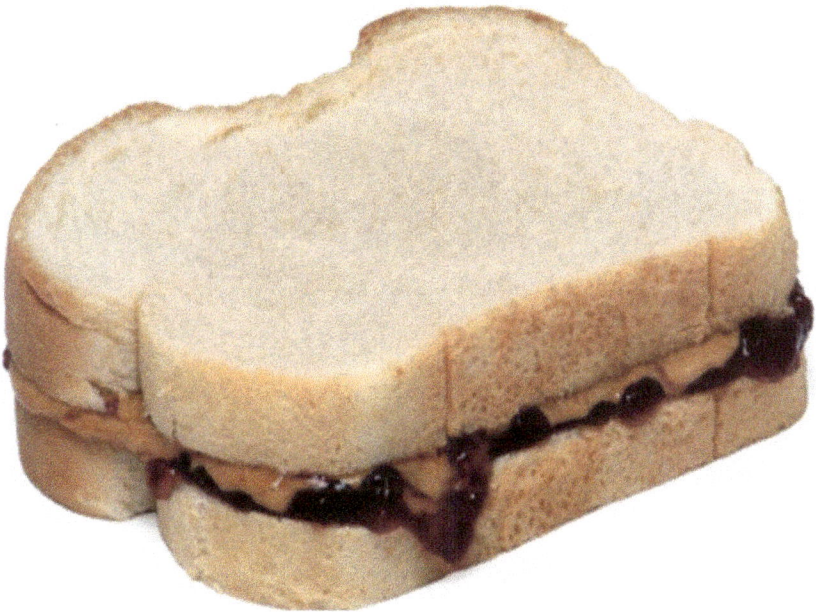

If I had not been able to get grandpa to wake up then I would have had to dial **9-1-1** on the phone to get help.

The **EMS** workers would have arrived in an ambulance. They would have checked his sugar level with their **glucometer**. If it was too low they would have given him a special sugar solution in his veins to get his sugar up quickly.

If his sugar was too high then they would have given him a salty solution called **saline** in his veins. That would reduce the sugar in his body.

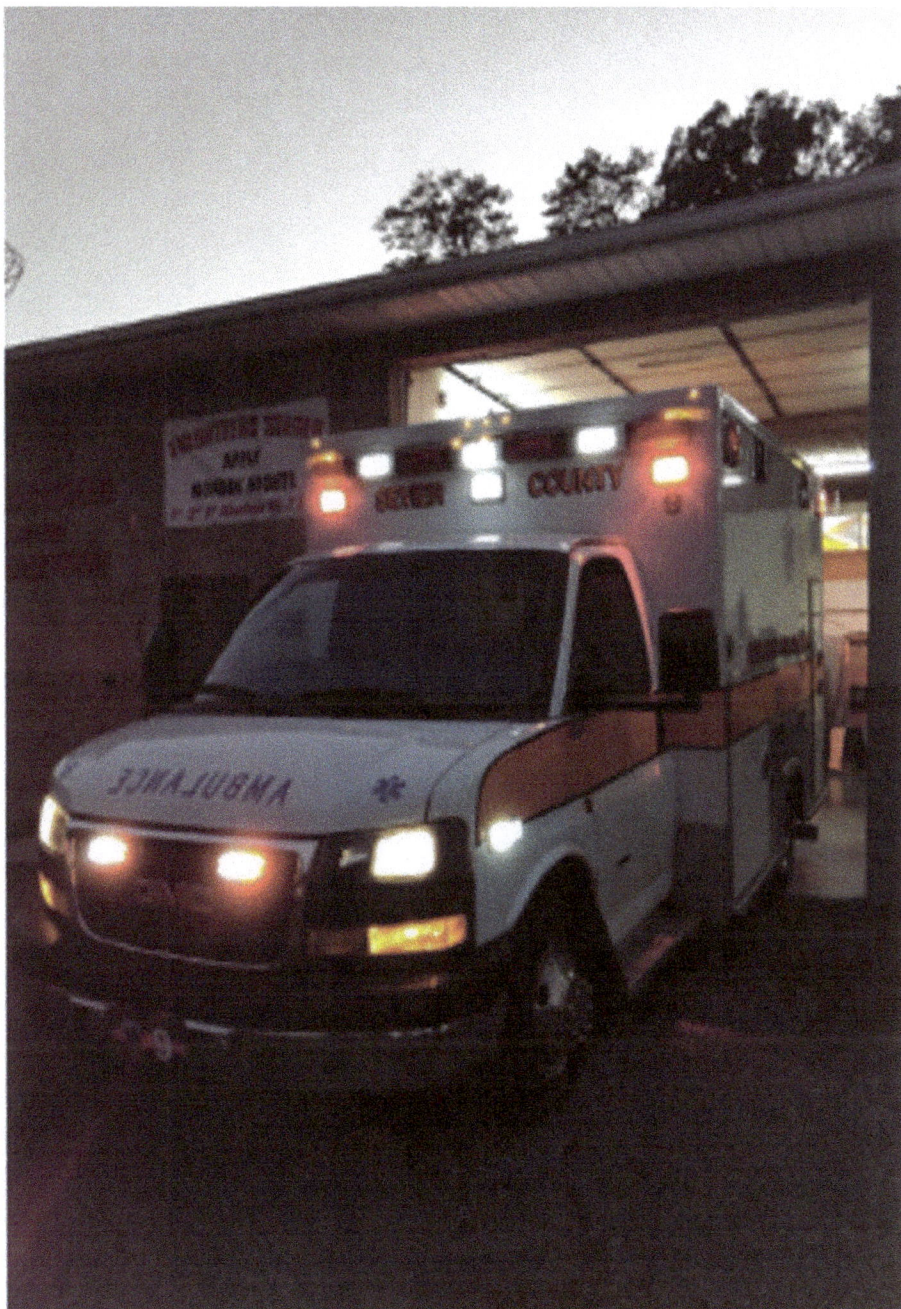

Always remember that medical items, like **glucometers** and needles, are not toys. They should never be played with. You should never bother a diabetic's **insulin**. And you should never attempt to give them **insulin** on your own. That should only be done by an adult or a medical professional.

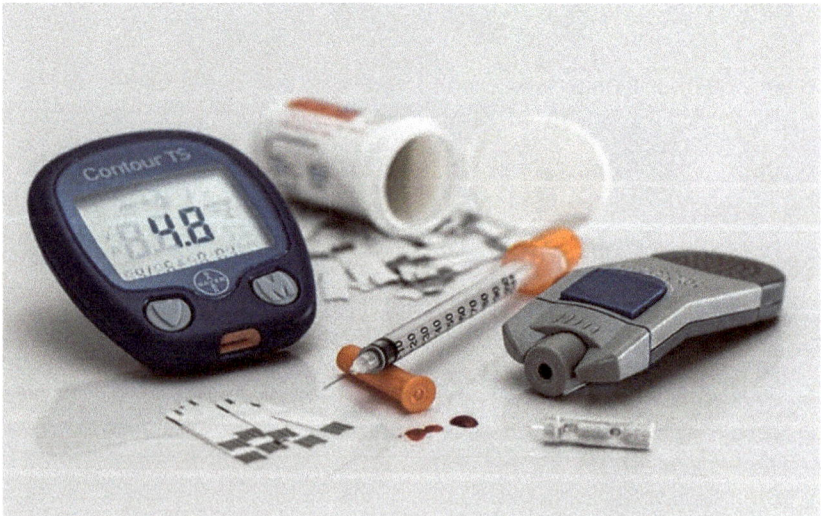

911 should never be called as part of a game. You should only dial **911** for a true emergency, such as not being able to wake up someone.

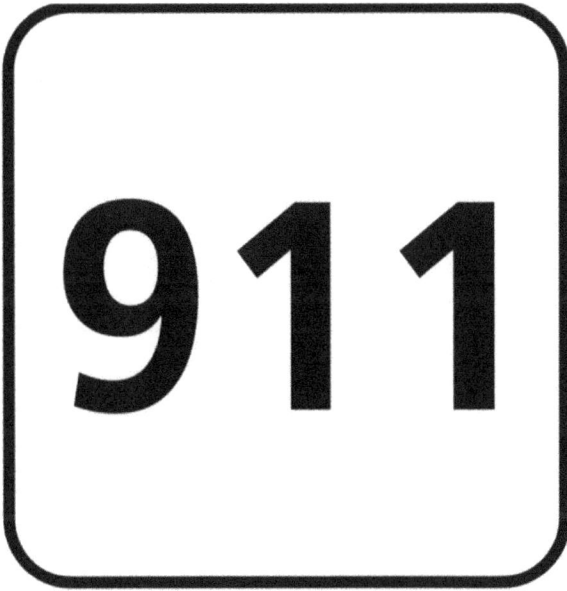

Always stay on the phone with the **911** operator until he or she tells you to hang up or until the **ambulance** or **First Responders** arrive.

You will need to tell the **911** operator what your emergency is, your name, address, and possibly your phone number so they can get help to you right away.

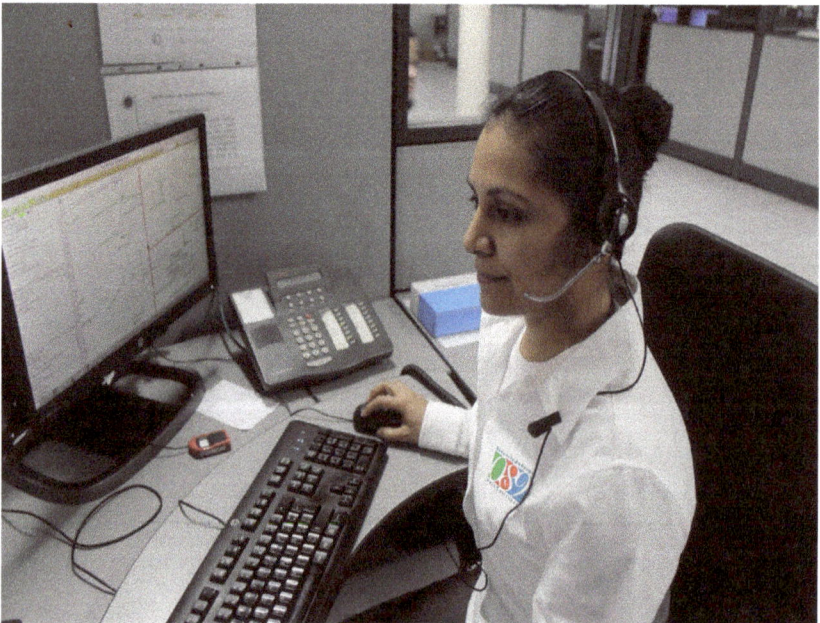

I'm very glad my grandpa, grandma, and mommy showed me how to help my grandpa when his sugar is low. Now I can help my grandpa stay alive and well.

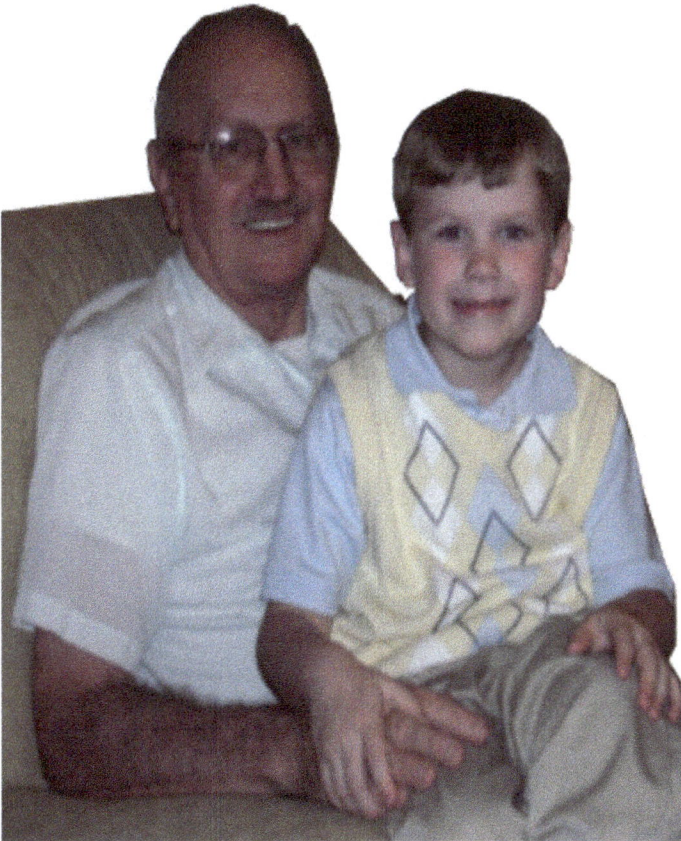

Symptoms of Hyperglycemia

(High blood sugar)

- Increased thirst
- Headache
- Trouble concentrating
- Blurred vision
- Frequent urination
- Feeling tired and weak often
- Weight loss (over period of time)
- Blood sugar reading over 180mg/dL

Symptoms of Hypoglycemia

(Low blood sugar level)

- Confusion
- Dizziness or lightheadedness
- Trembling or feeling shaky
- Excessive hunger
- Headache
- Irritability
- Pounding or racing heart or irregular heartbeat
- Pale skin
- Excessive sweating
- Weakness and fatigue
- Anxiety
- Poor coordination/unsteadiness
- Poor concentration or mental confusion
- Numbness or tingling in or around mouth and tongue
- Passing out/fainting

- Coma/unresponsiveness
- Dry mouth
- Nausea/vomiting
- Blurred vision
- Slurred Speech

Glossary

Ambulance – A vehicle that can be a van or box-shaped truck that has a cot to carry a patient on and has medical equipment to treat patients having a medical emergency. It has emergency lights and a siren to quickly respond to emergencies and get patients to a hospital quickly.

Carbohydrates – foods that are high in starch and/or sugar, such as potatoes, rice, pasta, candy, cakes, and pies.

Diabetes – an illness where the pancreas does not produce enough insulin to remove sugar from the blood and kidneys.

Diabetic - A person with diabetes.

Diabetic Coma – A situation where a diabetic person falls into a very deep sleep that is caused when a diabetic's blood sugar level is dangerously high or dangerously low.

EMS – Emergency Medical Services. These people are trained on what to do in case of a medical emergency and can transport a person to the hospital. They can be Advanced Emergency Medical Technicians or Paramedics.

First Responders – Men and women who are medically trained in first aid and CPR who often respond with the fire department or rescue squad.

Glucometer – A small hand held machine that tells how much sugar is in the blood.

Hyperglycemia – A condition where there is too much glucose (sugar) in the bloodstream.

Hypoglycemia – A condition where there is too little glucose (sugar) in the bloodstream.

Insulin – A hormone naturally produced in the pancreas that helps the body use carbohydrates and sugars. Also used as a treatment for diabetes.

9-1-1 – The number to call in case of an emergency to get in touch with EMS, Fire Department, or Police.

Saline – A salty, liquid sugar that is given through a needle in a vein.

For Further Reading

To find out more about Diabetes visit the American Diabetes Association at www.diabetes.org

You can also read more at www.webmd.com/diabetes and at

www.mayoclinic.org/diseases-conditions/diabetes

About the Author

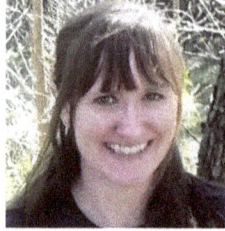

Leeza Wilson is a writer and licensed EMT Advanced in the state of Tennessee and a volunteer firefighter with Walden's Creek Volunteer Fire Department in Sevier County TN. She has always had a passion for the medical field. In 2007 she began working as an EMT with a county 911 service in South Carolina. In 2008 she began volunteering with Shepard Fire Department in Camden, South Carolina. She has a combined total of 10 years in the emergency services field.

When Leeza is not responding to emergency calls, she is writing poetry, fiction, and non-fiction for children and adults; running her publishing company; and spending time with her family.

Follow Me on Social Media

www.facebook.com/icanbeahero

www.twitter.com/leezatheauthor

www.instagram.com/leezatheauthor

www.facebook.com/leezatheauthor

To find out about upcoming releases in the series and other books published by Tsarina Press visit www.tsarinapress.com

Please Write a Review

Thank you for reading my book. It is my deepest wish that you had a pleasant reading experience and found this book informative and useful. Whether you did or didn't, please feel free to get in touch and let me know what you thought. I love hearing from my readers and I always try my best to respond to emails from my fans. I value your honest feedback.

As any author will tell you, reviews are so very important in helping our books get noticed. Reviews help authors reach more readers by letting them know if a book is worth reading or not. So I rely a lot on reviews to help readers find my books and know if they're worthy of investing their time in to read. It only takes a couple of minutes to write a brief review of what you thought of the book. So if you can take a minute to write an honest review, I would greatly appreciate it, even if it's a negative review. All reviews matter, whether they're 1 star or 5 stars, a small essay or just one word. Reviews can be left on Goodreads or any digital store where the book is sold.

Thanks!

Leeza Wilson